Fat Burning Nutrition and Workout Guide

Food and Exercise Suggestions to Help You Burn Fat, Lose Weight and Get a Sexy Body

RON KNESS

Copyright © 2017 Ron Kness

All rights reserved.

ISBN-13: 978-1544778877

ISBN-10: 1544778872

Contents

Disclaimer

This publication is for informational purposes only and is not intended as medical advice. Medical advice should always be obtained from a qualified medical professional for any health conditions or symptoms associated with them.

Every possible effort has been made in preparing and researching this material. We make no warranties with respect to the accuracy, applicability of its contents or any omissions.

See your healthcare professional before starting any diet, health or exercise program!

Introduction

When you want to lose weight, you need to get your body moving and increase your metabolism. There are certain workouts that help to burn more fat, helping you to reach your goals much faster. Here are some of the top fat-burning workouts.

Quick Power Walks

It is no surprise that walking is one of the best workouts

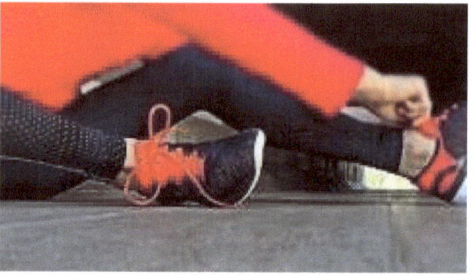

when you are trying to lose weight, but there are a lot of different forms of walking. If you are taking more casual walks for longer periods of time, you will keep your body moving and burn calories, but not burn as much fat. If you want to burn more fat, you need to increase the intensity. Instead of an hour-long casual walk, try a fast, power walk but for about 20-30 minutes.

Do Weights Before Cardio

Another effective method for burning fat is to do at least a few minutes of weight lifting before you do cardio. It is good to mix the two types of workouts regularly, but even on days when your only mission is to do some cardio, you should still be doing some weight lifting. People have found that when they do at least 10-15 minutes of weight lifting before stepping on the treadmill or elliptical, they lost weight more quickly and toned up at the same time.

Try Circuit Training

If you are not familiar with both cardio and weight lifting, then circuit training might be for you. Many fitness centers offer this as a class, or an area of the gym where each machine in a circuit is timed. This will make it a lot easier for you to do, without worrying about machines to do and for how long. It is an easy way to burn more fat at the gym and use a good amount of the machines without needing a personal training to show you how it's done.

Mix Up Your Workouts

This isn't a specific type of workout, but rather a method of exercising. IF you want to burn more fat while losing weight, then you don't want to do the same exact workout every single day. Instead, try mixing it up and adding in some yoga or Pilates, going for a hike instead of using the treadmill, or trying a new activity that gets your body moving, such as jumping in an indoor trampoline park. When you work different muscles of your body and have a different level of intensity, you start to burn more fat.

Cardio — How to Burn Fat On a Treadmill

You already know that cardio is one of the top ways to burn fat and drop weight. This has probably led you to look for different ways to get your cardio on and to burn fat at the same time. One of those methods is to use a treadmill. The misconception is that you can just get on the treadmill, set the timer, and get started. The truth to that misconception is that you will not see the results you want if you do just that. Here is how you turn your treadmill into a fat burning machine and get the results you want in shorter amounts of time.

Use the Incline Setting

The first thing you need to do is set the incline setting. You want to make sure that your incline is a challenge for you, but that it is not at such a high incline that it causes pain or injury. If you are just starting out with an incline, you may want to go with the first or second setting and then adjust as needed. Ideally, your treadmill will have several incline settings to choose from. One of these settings is an interval that mimics running outdoors in various terrains. Choose the one that is most comfortable for you. The treadmill will automatically adjust through your run to give you levels of incline to help you burn more calories. Or you can set it at a constant incline manually and it will stay there for the whole duration of your workout.

Know Your Target Heart Rate

Most treadmills come with a heart rate monitor built into them. Use the monitor. You may be inclined to avoid it or not bother, but if you want to burn the most fat and drop the weight you need to use the monitor.

For this, you will need to know your target heart rate. To figure this out, you need to know your maximum heart rate. The target heart rate during your workout should be around 60% of the max heart rate during cool down and warm up and then 70% to 80% during the run itself. Most treadmills will have at least a basic heart rate monitor, but more advanced options will let you put in your weight, height, and it will figure things out for you. This is vital to make sure you are getting the workout intensity you need. To figure out your maximum heart rate, take 220 minus your age. Then calculate the percentages from that figure.

Don't Hold On

One of the biggest mistakes people make when they are on the treadmill is to hold onto the bars. Don't hold onto the bars during the run. If you run hanging onto the bars, you will not be working your whole body. In fact, you will be holding back what you need to bring to the workout. By taking your hands off the bars you are now working your whole body – much the same if you were running outside. You are working on standing up straight, and running like you would outside. This intensifies the workout and helps you burn more fat.

By taking these three tips into account. You can ensure that you are burning the most calories and fat during your treadmill workout. Remember to start off at low levels of inclines and speed. Gradually work up your incline and run times; work up as you need to, so you can keep building the intensity and getting the results you want.

Weight Training

In terms of your workouts while losing weight, they should not be limited just to cardio. Weight training is really important for everyone, whether you are trying to burn fat or just be healthier overall. Here are some of the top benefits of adding weight training to your workout routine.

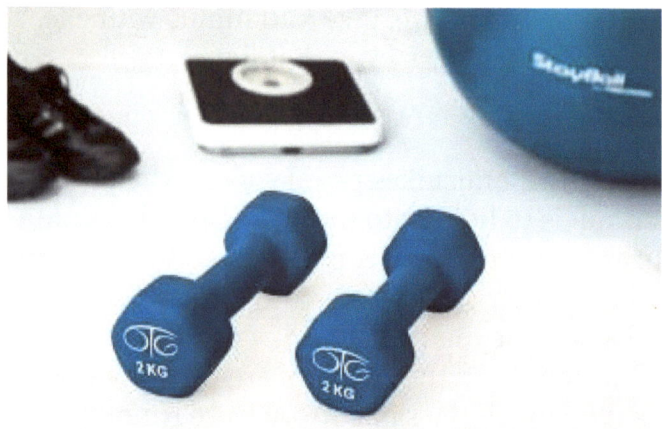

It Helps to Burn More Fat

Have you heard that muscle weighs more than fat? That is true, which is why many people look much leaner and wear smaller sizes in clothing, but the scale says they weigh more. This is because they have built up muscle through weight training, which is actually helping to burn more fat and calories. It takes more calories to support a pound of muscle than it does a pound of fat, hence the higher calorie burn of muscle. So they look thinner and more toned, but technically weigh more. This is why you shouldn't always pay attention to the scale, but work on weight training to look and feel better.

You Will Sleep Better

Weight training and working out your muscles gives you more energy during the day, but when it is time to rest and go to sleep, you will also sleep better. This is why after a day working hard at the gym, you practically fall asleep as soon as your head hits the pillow. With better sleep, you are also burning more fat and will have a better metabolism when you wake up, so this works great for you all around.

You Can Support Your Bones and Muscles

Nearly every part of your body benefits from weight training, including having better strength and support in your body for your muscles, bones, and tissue. Strength training helps to improve your bone density and will prevent bone loss as you age. Your muscles and tissue also get stronger, reducing potential injuries later in life. All of this is good news when you are trying to lose weight and want to avoid injuries that could keep you from your regular workouts.

It Gives a Better Quality of Life

As you can see from the benefits, weight training gives you a better quality of life. You avoid injury, lose weight faster and easier by burning more fat, and will just look and feel better overall. There are a lot of reasons to add weight training to your fitness routine and not many reasons to avoid doing it.

You don't have to spend hours every day working on weights either; try a simple circuit training session at your gym or some kettlebell videos that you can do right in your living room.

Burn More Fat With Weight Training

When you think of weight training, you may not think about burning fat. In fact, what you may think about is building muscle and toning up your arms or adding muscle weight. The trick to that is, most people who are new to weight training do not know that you have to burn fat to build the muscle which makes weight training ideal. If you are new to weight training, you may not know how to actually get started or how to make the weight training work for the fat burning you want to do.

Use the Right Weight

If you are new to weight training, then you want to make sure you are choosing the right weight from the start. Some gym professionals will tell you to start off with body weight first. This is ideal if you are not only new to weight training, but you are also considered obese. Think about this. If you are 100 pounds overweight, you are already carrying 100 pounds of weight lifting pressure. Use that and work it off. You can use a weightlifting bar for balance which adds a few more pounds, but mainly gives you something to work with for stability purposes. Finally, you get to add the weight. Start off with 10 pounds on each side of the bar and then work your way up to more as you get stronger.

Use the Right Form

There is nothing worse than working out and either injuring yourself or realizing that you are using the wrong form and you aren't burning as much body fat as you could be. The way to fix this is to find a professional and just make sure you are using the right form. A professional trainer will show you how to use the right form for the bar-based weights, the circuit weight training machines, and free weights.

Using the right form means you are getting the most out of the weight training, using the muscles under the fat, and burning the fat away properly and safely.

Circuit the Workout

Don't stick to just one form of weight or one exercise. For example, don't just do an arm day and do a few of the same exercises. Circuit your body. This means that you are doing a certain amount of reps for each focus-area exercise. So for arms, you would be working all aspects of your arms and chest. You would be doing five to ten reps on each section and then doing it again for three or more complete circuits. This helps your body relax in one area while you are working another, and the whole time you are burning the most fat possible.

These are the basic steps for burning fat when you are a newcomer to weight training. Overtime you may find that free weights work best for you or that circuit training works best. The key is to start off safe and start off with the right form.

Add These Cardio Workouts

Burning fat sounds great and easy, until you get into it. Once you have been working out for awhile, you may hit a moment where you just don't seem to be burning more fat or getting anywhere with the workouts. You may try to up the pace of your runs, change your weight amount on weight lifting, or any number of other things just to be at the same point. This means your body may be used to the workouts and you need to actually change the workouts. Here are some cardio workouts you can add to your routine to help you burn more fat and get back on track.

Spinning Class

One way that some people mix things up is by enrolling in a spinning class. Spinning classes take stationary bikes to the next level. The classes run from 30 minutes to 75 minutes. The idea behind these classes is to offer a high intensity constant moving workout. It works your quads, core, abs, arms, calves, and hamstrings. It can be a full body workout that burns a lot of calories which leads to fat burning as well. This is a high intensity method and is usually made for more intermediate and advanced workouts. Spinning can work off as much as 900 calories per session.

Indoor Rock Climbing

Okay, you may not think of rock climbing as a fat burning exercise, but you can bump up your fat burning by simply adding this to your routine. As you climb, you are working your entire body. You are lifting your bodyweight, moving your arms and legs, and you are working your core. This burns calories. The higher you climb, the more intense the fat burning becomes. If you are new to indoor rock climbing, you can start with a beginner wall and them move up. This type of exercise can keep you busy and engaged for several years before you run out of what you can do indoors and then can move it outdoors if you like.

You can add one or all three of these to routine. You will see an increase in fat burning and you can keep up the rotation of your normal workout routine alongside this new routine.

Yoga and Pilates

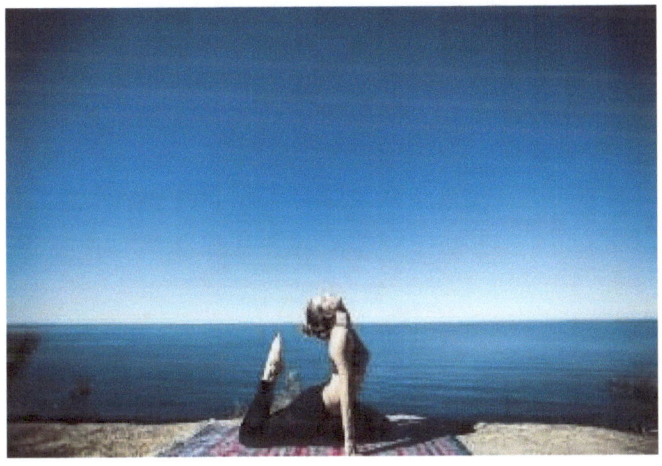

One of the top exercises recommended for beginners and advanced users alike is yoga or Pilates. These exercises have several full body benefits and the added benefit of helping you burn fat. You may be wondering what types of yoga or Pilates actually help you burn the most fat and get a full body workout. The truth is, there are several that offer a full workout, full body benefit. Here are just a few to consider.

Hot Yoga

Hot Yoga is one of the leading yoga methods that offers a full body workout, cleansing of toxins, and fat burning exercise. This form of yoga, also known as Bikram Yoga, offers up to a 700 calorie burn depending on the intensity of the class and time of that class. During this yoga session you will notice a few things that set it apart from other yoga classes. The first is the temperature. Hot yoga classes are set at 104 degrees in the room. This helps you to sweat more which purges more toxins from your body during the workout. The humidity is also set high for the room. You will work through over 60 different motions through the workout.

By the end, you will have worked your entire body as well as built your cardio and purged your system of toxins.

Pilates

There is a fine line in the yoga community with half the people stating that Pilates is not real yoga while the other half stating that it is yoga just in a different from. Pilates stands out because it uses different instruments during the workout. For example, you may use a Pilates machine that offers resistance or you may use a Pilates ball. The accessories are there to help stabilize you and help you get your workout to the next level. If you want something that incorporates traditional yoga but adds a twist on the process, then this may be ideal for you.

Kundalini Yoga

Kundalini yoga is a cardio-based yoga that works your entire body while working on your cardio. This combination allows you to burn more fat and helps you to get leaner muscle mass as well. There are no special accessories in Kundalini. Kundalini requires your body, body weight resistance, and your mind. Ideally, if you are looking for a form of yoga that will burn fat and give you a full body workout while helping you with meditation and body awareness then this is it. Kundalini focuses on full body awareness through meditation and body movement.

These are only three of the yoga and Pilates options that will help you burn fat and drop the weight. You can increase the intensity of each one of these workouts by adding more time, taking intense training to work on your form, or by just adding more days of these yoga routines into your weekly rotation.

Yoga Poses That Burn More Fat

If you are looking to burn more fat with your workouts, just
doing cardio and weight
training might not get
you to where you want to
be. Another good option
is to mix up your
workouts and add in
some yoga. Here are
some of the best yoga

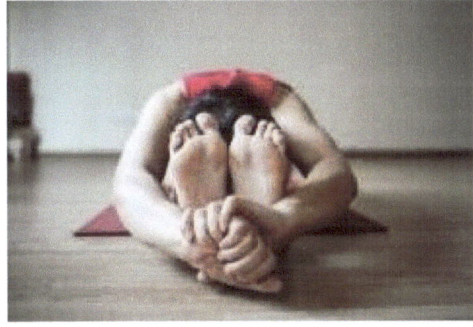

poses for burning more fat and helping you to lose weight.

Down Dog Split

This yoga pose is similar to a down dog pose, but it is going
to have a slight variation called a split. You will start the yoga
pose by getting into the downward dog position, then move
one of your legs up, which helps to open your hip at the same
time. Do this while inhaling a breath. Then when you let out
the air by exhaling, you will round your knee close to your
nose, pulling up your leg to your abdomen. Now release it
and repeat with the other side. Keep doing this for about 10
reps on each leg and you will burn a lot of fat and calories
from the movements.

Plank

A simple plank is a yoga pose that packs a lot of power and is
great for burning more fat. Planks look simple when you see
other people do them until you attempt them yourself. It
really is a full-body workout that you can do just about
anywhere. A plank is done by getting on your hands and
knees on the ground, then lifting your body with your hands
flat on the ground and your toes resting on the ground.

The rest of your body is lifted off the ground, from your arms down to your legs.

Wheel

The wheel yoga pose is more of an advanced pose but will also work out your entire body and help you to burn more fat. You will start this pose on your back laying on your yoga mat, bending your knees and keeping your feet off the ground similar to starting a sit-up. Your elbows should be bent, with your hands on the sides of your head. Now start moving your hands and feet at the same time while lifting your hips. This tuck motion looks like an abdominal crunch, but you are focusing on your breathing the entire time.

Try taking a yoga class like hot yoga to burn even more calories and lose weight while doing the poses.

Mix It Up With Circuit Training

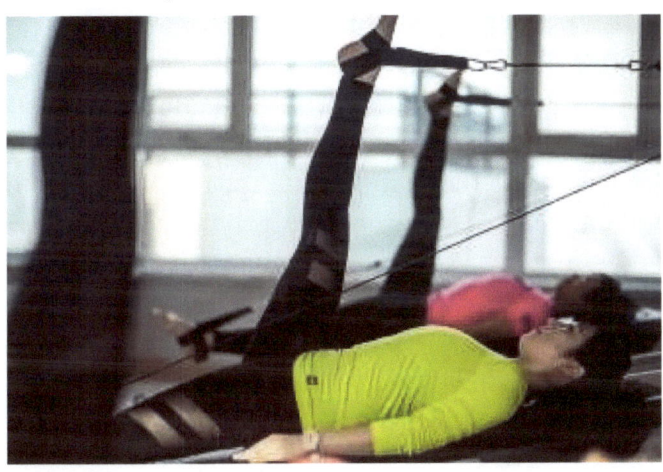

When you go the gym, you may see a small area of machines that are lined up in two rows sitting back to back. This is a circuit training station and is one way that you can mix up your workout and burn more fat. If you have never used a circuit training method, there are some things that you should know and consider before getting started. Here are those common considerations and what you need to know about each one of them.

The Proper Circuit

If you have never worked these machines, you may not know what the proper circuit is. The truth is you should start at one end or the other and work your way around the circuit of machines. Each machine works a different part of the body and each has a set of weights for you to set the right weight for your workout. In other words, there is no proper circuit or right machine to start off with. Just pick one of the end machines and get started. The idea is to work through each machine at least three times. You can increase the weight during each round or leave it where it is.

Weight Level

Once you get started, you will need to set the weight to the right level. You want a weight that is intense enough that it makes each rep worth the time and works your muscles. You also don't want it to be so high that you end up causing injury to yourself. Ideally, you will want to start with a lower weight, 10 to 20 pounds, and work up. You want to have some resistance with the weights. If the workout is too easy, you aren't going to get the benefit that you are looking for. If it is too hard, you will cause damage to your body. Start slow, work up the levels. Also, keep in mind that you can change the weight for legs and arms. For example, if you have more strength in your legs you may want a higher weight for your legs than your arms.

Don't Focus on Cardio

One of the mistakes that people make with circuit training is trying to focus on the cardio aspect. Ignore the cardio for now. Though you may not feel like you are getting your heart rate up or that you are getting what you need, your muscles are getting the workout they need. What you need to do is focus on the circuit, pay attention to your body, and take the warning signs your body is giving you if there is an issue that could lead to injury. If you feel to strained, lower the weight intensity.

These are just three of the considerations to keep in mind with your circuit training workout when you are trying to mix it up with your normal workout routine. Remember to meet with a professional to check your form as well. If your form is off, your workout will be as well.

Fat-Burning Workouts for a Flat Tummy

Just about everyone wants a flatter tummy, but just losing weight isn't always going to get you there. You also need to add certain workouts that help you to target the right areas. These workouts are perfect for getting a flat tummy.

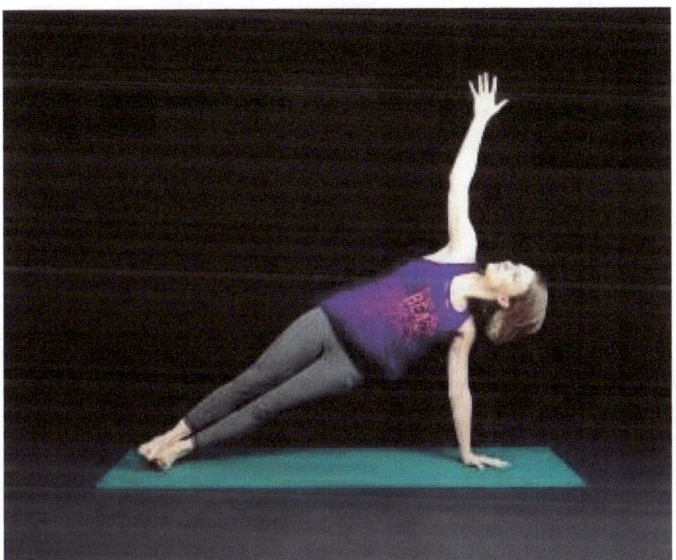

Side Plank

You already know that a regular plank is great for burning fat and is awesome for your core, arms and legs, but for a flat tummy, a side plank is even better. This isn't the easiest move to pull off, and does take practice. But the more often you try it, the stronger you get, and the better you will be. Plus for every practice session, you are working out muscles that burn fat and flatten your tummy more and more.

The side plank is done by lying on one side and resting on your elbow, then putting the opposite hand on the other shoulder or on the hip. Hold it for a few seconds, then switch to the other side.

Reverse Plank

Another plank exercise that is good for a flat tummy and will burn more fat is the reverse plank, sometimes referred to as a plank hover. This is also similar to a plank but with a few modifications that help to work more muscles. Instead of your face close to the ground, you are doing it the other direction. You can start it by sitting on the ground with your feet facing forward. You want to put your hands on the ground and try to lift your body up to where your hips are a little bit off the ground. Hold it for a few seconds and release. Try a few repetitions if you can.

Alligator Drag

This last move is not a plank, but it works just as many muscles and is perfect for getting a flat tummy. You are going to work out your entire core, plus you will work on upper and lower body muscles at the same time. You need a good amount of ground to use, up to 20 yards as you are going to be moving ahead of you. You also need something to help you slide across the floor, like a plastic bag or towel. Get into a full pushup on the ground, then put the objects under your feet. You are going to walk and slide forward, then walk backward.

Fat-Burning Meal Ideas

Breakfast

As you know, breakfast is one of the most important meals of the day. It keeps you full and gives you energy, which is important when you want to become a fat-burning machine. Here are some fat-burning breakfast ideas to try out.

Blueberry Oatmeal Pancakes

Here is a super simple way to have a filling breakfast that burns more fat and calories, while also being delicious. Just because you are trying to eat healthier and are careful about your nutrition, doesn't mean you can't still have pancakes. You just might want to go from traditional buttermilk pancakes with butter and syrup, and instead have this healthier alternative. These pancakes are made with some of the regular pancake ingredients, like vanilla extract and eggs. Then you will use low-fat cottage cheese, rolled oats, and blueberries. For the top, combine yogurt with maple syrup.

Fruit Smoothie

Smoothies are easy to make in the morning when you need a grab-and-go option, but they can also be really good for you and contain fat burning ingredients.

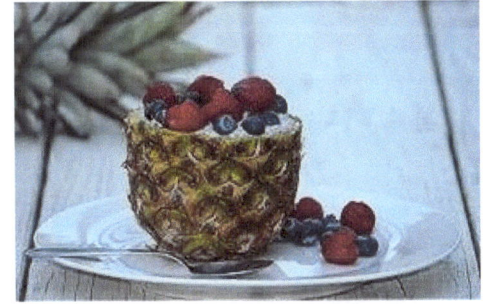

The trick here is to include ingredients that are known to burn fat, like high fiber fruits such as strawberries and mango, low-fat dairy products, and greens like kale or spinach. You can make a fruit smoothie with tropical fruits like pineapple and mango, or go traditional with a mixed berry smoothie of strawberries, blueberries, and raspberries. Also remember that you can use frozen bananas instead of ice, which make the smoothie cold but also add some creaminess to it.

Almond Butter Toast

Here is another fast and easy breakfast that fills you up and burns more fat at the same time. Use whole grain bread for your toast, which on its own is great for fat burning. You will then use some almond butter on top instead of regular butter or peanut butter. On top of that, add some sliced banana. For more flavor, you can drizzle some raw honey on top, but it isn't necessary and that adds more sugar that you might not want. One big slice of almond butter toast with banana slices can be under 300 calories, so it is a good size for a breakfast.

Egg Scramble

Eggs are a great source of protein and provide some excellent fat burning properties. A simple way to make eggs in the morning is to scramble up some eggs with a little low-fat cheese and your choice of chopped veggies. Some good options are bell peppers, onions, tomatoes, and mushrooms.

Lunch

When it comes time for lunch, you want to keep that metabolism up by choosing ingredients that will help you to keep burning more fat for the rest of the day.

These lunches provide a good balance of nutrients that are going to help you stay on track around midday.

Grilled Chicken and Veggies

It doesn't get much simpler than this! You can make a grilled chicken dinner the night before and save leftovers for lunch, or grill some chicken cutlets, slice them up, and put them in individual containers for lunches. You can also try using a rotisserie chicken and cutting it up for your lunches. Choose your choice of veggies for this healthy lunch, such as going with summer veggies like corn, squash, and zucchini, or you can add a southwestern flair by adding in some bell peppers, black beans, corn, and tomatoes. There is really a lot of room for customization with this type of healthy, fat burning lunch.

Turkey and Avocado Sandwich

This sandwich can be made either as a simple cold sandwich, or into a melt like a grilled cheese. IF you want to do a melt, you can make it an open-faced sandwich on the grill and use just one slice of cheese on one slice of bread. The other 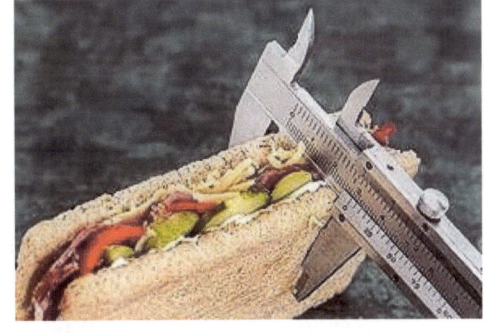 half of the bread can contain the lunch meat and avocado, plus any other veggies you want. When both slices are heated up and browned, remove them from the grill and press them together. It is super easy! You can customize this with any deli meat or veggies you want.

Quinoa Salad

Here is another healthy and delicious lunch that is light enough for a quick lunch, but is also filling. Quinoa is a type of grain that contains a lot of protein and iron, plus can be combined with just about anything. You can have just quinoa and chopped veggies, add in some lean protein, or top a bed of lettuce and veggies with the cooked quinoa. It is very versatile with a mild nutty flavor that goes great with a lot of other seasonings and herbs. Plus, as a whole grain, quinoa and the veggies you mix it with are going to be perfect for burning more fat. If you make quinoa for dinner and have some leftover, add it to a container to use for a lunch later in the week.

Dinner

Speaking of dinner, you most likely aren't just feeding yourself, but your family as well. If you are trying to lose weight, this can be difficult because you don't want to make two separate meals. Luckily, there are some healthy and delicious dinners that your family will love, but that also burn more fat and help you to stay on track.

Salmon, Veggies, and Nuts

Salmon is one of the best types of protein you can eat. It is easy to cook, low in fat and calories, and delicious for everyone in the family. It will be light enough for you and help to burn fat, but your family will enjoy the delicious maple flavor. You can use maple syrup and vinegar plus a little Dijon mustard to make a marinade for the salmon that really brings out its flavors. Combine this salmon with your choice of veggies, whether you go with green beans and mushrooms, broccoli and cauliflower medley, or a side salad.

Top the salad with some chopped walnuts and almonds for crunch and added nutrients.

White Bean Chili

The reason this is a good dinner is because your family gets to enjoy chili with their own side, like their favorite type of rolls, while you get something hearty and nutritious. The white bean chili doesn't use any meat in it unless you want to add some turkey or chicken, which makes it on the lighter side. It contains beans, lentils, and spices that burn more fat, like the white beans, quinoa, and some turmeric and ginger in there. You can add in any other spices or veggies that you want. Serve it alone or with a side salad.

Turkey Burgers

If you are looking for a high-protein dinner that is going to fill you up, but also make your family happy, try making some turkey burgers. Ground turkey when using the right seasonings, doesn't taste that different from beef. Your spouse and kids probably won't even miss the beef! However, if you want lighter burgers but keep some of that beef flavor in, try doing half turkey and half beef. Combine it together and place them on a skillet or grill them up. Skip the cheese and mayonnaise, and instead use mustard which burns fat, along with plenty of vegetables and lettuce on the burger. Serve it with any healthy side dish your family will enjoy.

Snacks

If your mission is to lose weight, then burning fat should be at the top of your list. One way to do this is by picking some good fat-burning snacks. The following snacks are really easy to grab and take with you, but also burn lots of fat and get you on the path of weight loss.

Figs

Figs are a type of fruit that not many people are familiar with. They have a lot of fiber, are sweet like some of your other favorite fruits, and can fill you up quickly. Figs help you to curb your cravings and reduce your appetite by filling you up, but they also help to burn fat at a faster rate. They are ideal when you are trying to find an easy snack you can just grab on your way out the door, but something light that is going to help you burn fat during the day. You can get either fresh or dried figs.

Kale Chips

Another type of snack that is healthy and will also help to burn more fat is kale chips. These can be purchased in a health food store, or you can easily make them yourself. By making them on your own, you reduce the sodium and other additives, plus you save quite a bit of money. All you need to do is cut kale into smaller pieces, put it on a cookie sheet and drizzle olive oil with some sea salt and pepper. Bake them for about 15 minutes or until crisp and store in a plastic bag or container. These are filling and super low in fat, plus kale is great for burning more fat.

Pistachios

In terms of nuts, pistachios are one of the most delicious, and also happen to be one of the best options when you want to burn more fat. Sure, they might be a little higher in calories than what you are used to, but this is healthy fat. Eating them as a snack keeps the carbs low and your protein and energy high. Put them in portion bags that you can quickly grab and throw in your purse or lunch bag on your way out the door.

This will prevent you from over-indulging in them, but make sure you always have a healthy snack with you.

Avocado

Avocado is another fat-burning food that is easy to enjoy as a snack. Open up an avocado and just sprinkle some salt on it, or you can enjoy it mashed with some salsa, similar to guacamole. Dip some veggies in it and you're good to go.

Fruits and Veggies

For a well-balanced diet, you need to have plenty of fruits and veggies in addition to your lean protein and whole grains. Luckily, they are not only low in fat and nutritious, but many of them actually help to burn more fat.

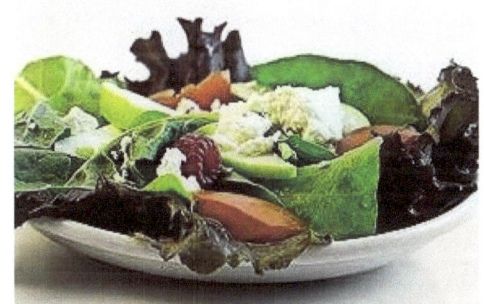

High Fiber Fruits

There are many fruits that are nutritious and good for, which most of them containing vitamins and minerals that will be good overall. However, not all fruits are equal in terms of how well they burn fat and help you lose weight. When you want to burn more fat with your fruit, look for ones that have a lot of fiber, as this is going to help fill you up, improve your digestion, plus burn more of your body fat. To start with, have more apples. These are low in sugar, high in flavor and high in fiber.

You can also have your fill of berries, which are loaded with antioxidants and burn fat as well. These also happen to be low-carb approved, so if you are on a low carb diet, you can still enjoy them. Go for strawberries and blueberries first, then raspberries and other types. Avocadoes often get confused with being a vegetable, but they are actually fruit. They also boost your metabolism and are a good healthy fat to enjoy. Finally, add grapefruit to the list, which helps you to burn fat and has loads of vitamin C.

Nutrient Dense Vegetables

Now for the best fat burning vegetables. You definitely want to add as many veggies to your diet as you can, opting for frozen or fresh whenever possible. Try to avoid canned vegetables as they typically have a lot of sodium that you don't want or need.

The vegetables with the best fat burning abilities are those that contain the most nutrients. To start with, try adding more chili peppers and bell peppers to your diet. They have a high amount of fiber and plenty of vitamin C and 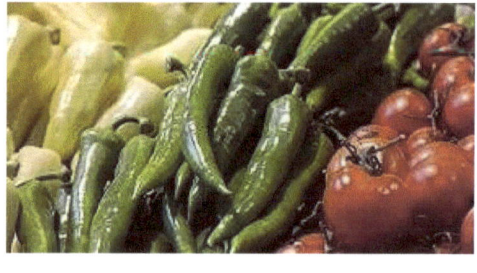 vitamin A. Broccoli is also high in fiber and contains the same nutrients.

Kale is one of the best leafy greens to add to your diet, helping to burn fat and providing you with calcium, protein, and fiber. Don't forget about lentils, which are going to help improve your digestion and improve weight loss at the same time. Luckily, all of these veggies are delicious and easy to add to your meals.

Burn More Fat With These Smoothies

Burning fat includes a good balance of diet and exercise. In terms of your nutrition, smoothies are a great place to burn fat. They often include fruits and other ingredients that help to give you energy and boost your metabolism. Give some of these smoothie recipes a try.

Mango Smoothie

If you like mango fruit, then you will love this fun smoothie! It only uses a few simple ingredients and is very easy to make. Plus, it includes multiple ingredients that help to burn fat, including the mango, lime juice, and avocado. Don't worry; it won't taste like a vegetable. The sweetness of the fruit far outweighs the flavor of the avocado. Just get out your blender and add mango pieces, a mashed avocado, vanilla yogurt, and lime juice. You can add a little bit of sugar if you want, but it is not needed. Finish it off with some ice or half a frozen banana.

Citrus Smoothie

You can also use your favorite citrus fruits and combine them with ice and your choice of dairy product to make a sweet, creamy smoothie that helps you to lose weight. Some citrus fruits that usually go good are lemons, oranges, and grapefruit, but go ahead and use any combination of fruits you have at home. You want to make it creamy with a little bit of yogurt and some skim milk. You can use flavored yogurt like lemon, or just plain fat-free yogurt. Add some ice and a little flaxseed or chia seed for added fat burning potential.

Berry Smoothie

Berries are at the top of the list for fruits that help to burn more fat and calories. Strawberries in particular contain a lot of antioxidants and are high in fiber, which helps you to increase your fat burning. You can make a simple smoothie with strawberries and other berries, with skim milk, yogurt, and flaxseed oil. For a thicker smoothie, add some oats to it.

Blueberry Smoothie

Another version of the berry smoothie is one that contains blueberries. This provides a slightly different flavor, but the same health benefits of a strawberry or mixed berry smoothie. Plus, blueberries contain a lot of nutrients and antioxidants that make it a popular superfood. Blueberries taste great just with milk or yogurt and ice, but you can also add in raw honey or frozen banana instead of ice.

Try out your own combinations using these and other fruits.

Refreshing Fat-Burning Drinks

When you choose what you want to drink as you are working on losing weight, you should also be thinking about what could burn the most fat. This is when you are going to go from occasional weight loss to continued weight loss. Here are some fat burning drinks to try out.

Green Tea

If you choose just one drink aside from water, it should be green tea. This is so good for you, can easily be flavored with honey or skim milk, and provides a lot of energy. Green tea also has tons of other health benefits, like improving your skin, increasing your metabolism, and helping to clean out your system. Green tea also happens to contain a lot of antioxidants, and most varieties are caffeine-free. Try to have at least one cup of green tea, but feel free to enjoy as many cups as you like.

Skim Milk

While there is no reason you can't have whole milk, skim milk does tend to be a better beverage when you are losing weight and burning fat. Skim milk is going to be lower in fat and calories, so you can get the much needed calcium and other nutrients from milk, without actually affecting your weight loss in a negative way. Calcium is really important when losing weight or trying to get healthy in general, so enjoy a little skim milk with breakfast or in your smoothie.

Infused Water

You probably already know how important water is, but think about certain versions of water that can aid you in your fat burning efforts. Infused water has fruit and veggies in it, many of which are also going to help to burn more fat and help you lose weight. Plus, when you drink ice cold water, that can help to give you energy and speed up your metabolism. Start drinking at least 8-10 eight-ounce glasses of water a day, preferably ice cold water and try to make some of them infused water.

Vegetable Juice

Another great beverage to have when you want to burn more fat is vegetable juice. This should not be something you get in a bottle or can, but vegetable juice you make for yourself at home. Get a juicer and juice veggies like celery, carrots, kale, 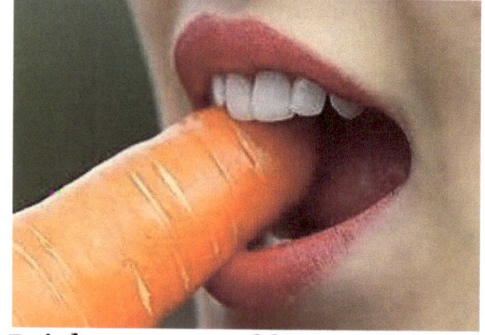 spinach, and many others. Drink your vegetable juice cold and before a meal to burn more calories and fat even while eating the meal. Plus it will help fill you up before you eat a meal.

Infused Water Recipes For Weight Loss

Infused water is a type of water that includes fruits, vegetables, and herbs that are infused in the water for added flavor. It is easy to make and is a great way to use produce without actually eating it. The following infused water recipes are great for losing weight and burning more fat.

Apple and Cinnamon

Both apple sand cinnamon are good ingredients to use when you want to burn more fat. Cold water also happens to be good for burning fat and calories and increasing your energy levels throughout the day. So make this infused water the night before, keep the pitcher in the fridge, and you will be ready to turn yourself into a fat-burning machine with delicious water. All you need to do is add some sliced apples to the bottom of the pitcher, being sure no seeds are present, then 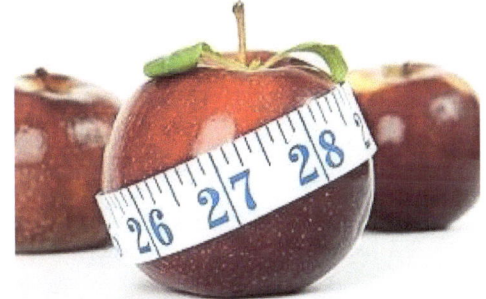 one cinnamon stick. This is much better than powdered sugar for water so it doesn't cause clogs or clumps in the water. Let it sit overnight with filtered water and that's it!

Berry and Lemon

For this infused water, you can use any berries you want. Most berries are good for burning fat and contain a lot of antioxidants. Both blueberries and strawberries also happen to be superfoods, which is even better for you. You can also try other types of berries, like raspberries and blackberries. To the berries at the bottom of the pitcher, add some lemon slices as well for more detox potential. Fill it with filtered water and leave in the fridge overnight. You can also add some ice on top of the fruit to release the flavors and keep the water nice and cold.

Watermelon and Mint

Many infused waters also contain herbs, which provide more flavor and nutrients at the same time. This infused water is super simple and tastes mostly like the watermelon slices you add, but you are also going to have some mint in there. Try to use a seedless watermelon, and use slices that don't have a lot of rind on them. This allows you to get as much fruit flavor as possible. Add some muddled mint at the bottom, cover with ice, then fill with water.

When making your infused water, try to use fresh and organic fruit whenever possible. You can also add slices of vegetables and herbs as needed for more nutrients and added flavor.

Important Nutrients, Herbs and Spices For Weight Loss

When it comes to weight loss, it isn't just about exercising as much as you can or 'dieting'. You also want to focus on proper nutrition, which includes the vitamins, minerals, and other nutrients that help you live a healthier life, while also burning fat. Here are some of the top nutrients to add to your diet.

Whole Grains

The first type of nutrient you should add to your diet if you want to start losing more weight is whole grains. These are recommended for many different types of diets, even some low-carb diets. Whole grains are good for you, not heavily processed, and 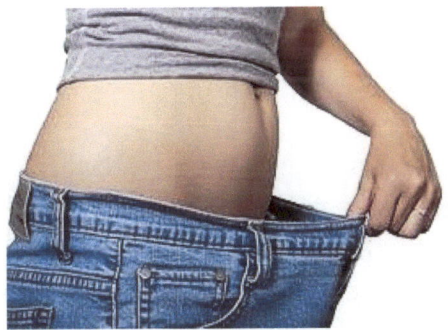 contain a lot of important nutrients like a high amount of fiber. You definitely want more fiber in your diet if you are going to burn more fat and calories. Some good sources of whole grains and high fiber are brown rice, whole grain breads, and oatmeal.

Vitamin D and Calcium

Both vitamin D and calcium are important when you are getting healthy and losing weight. These nutrients help to burn more fat by building muscle mass and helping to protect your muscles and bones as you age.

Both of these nutrients are often found together in dairy products, so those are good to add to your regular diet. You can go for fat-free or low-fat dairy products if you are watching your overall amount of fat and calories each day as these still contain the important nutrients you need.

Iron

Another nutrient you can try to get more of and burn fat at the same time is iron. Iron is often found in lean protein, vegetables, and lentils. Many people know that if they have more turkey and lean cuts of beef, they will get plenty of iron and protein at the same time, but they often forget about their lentils and veggies. Some good sources of iron include leafy greens like spinach and kale, plus your different lentils. Both of these together can be added to a low-fat chili or soup recipe, which is filling and is loaded with essential nutrients.

Start thinking of ways to add these types of foods to your diet, from making a vegetable and lentil soup for a light and filling dinner, to having more low-fat dairy products like smoothies or yogurt with fruit as a healthy snack. As long as you know what to add, it is easy to have a healthy diet that also helps you to burn more fat.

Add These Herbs and Spices to Your Meals

As you start meal planning to help you on your weight loss journey, you should also think about how you season your dishes. Herbs and spices don't just add flavor, but can actually help you to burn more fat. Here are some that you definitely want to include.

Ginseng

One of the best herbs that can help you burn more fat is ginseng. It burns fat by naturally speeding up your metabolism and helping to boost your energy levels. When your metabolism gets a nice boost, you are able to burn fat and calories at a more rapid pace. Plus, the extra energy makes you more motivated to exercise, also increasing how much fat you burn. You can get ginseng extract or get supplements that are really easy to take, so you don't even have to add it to your meals.

Cinnamon

Who doesn't love a little cinnamon? Luckily, not only is it delicious, cinnamon is good for you! It contains a lot more nutrients than you might imagine and can also help to boost your metabolism. Cinnamon helps with lowering blood sugar from diabetes and can even help with your cholesterol levels. So when you want to add some flavor to your coffee, sprinkle a little cinnamon on top. You can also make a delicious smoothie that tastes like dessert by combining skim or soy milk with apples and cinnamon on top.

Mustard

Yes, mustard is good for you! This spice is often used on fattening foods like hot dogs, but it doesn't have to be. You can add mustard spice or mustard seeds to a lot of different foods and side dishes that aren't bad for you. You may want to make a sandwich with lean meats, veggies, and whole grain brain, then flavor it with a little mustard. Also try dipping some of your favorite veggies in mustard. You will be amazed by how good this can be.

Turmeric

Turmeric is becoming popular as a spice because it tastes great and is extremely healthy. As a superfood, turmeric provides loads of nutrients that help you to be healthier overall, but also to burn fat and improve your weight loss efforts. It tastes similar to curry, so if you like a little kick to your veggie or rice dishes, sprinkle some turmeric in there. There are many different easy and healthy ways to use turmeric in your cooking.

Final Thoughts

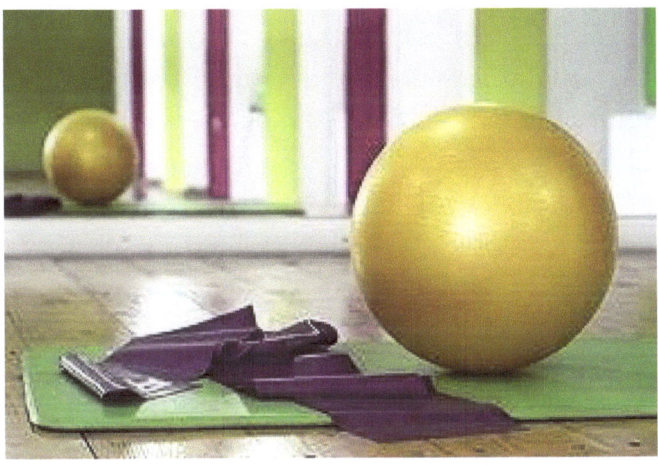

In order to lose weight, you want to become a fat burning machine. There are many ways to do that, most of which are not difficult at all. Here are some things you can do every day that will help you to burn more fat.

Increase Your Protein

One great way to start burning more fat on a regular basis is to eat more foods that contain protein. With more protein in your diet, you are going to start increasing your energy. Higher energy, as you know, also means a higher metabolic rate, which helps you to burn more fat and calories. Protein also helps to build lean muscle, which can also help to burn more fat throughout the day. Some good options for lean protein are turkey and chicken, nuts, and some veggies.

Stop Skipping Breakfast

Breakfast still remains the most important meal of the day, so if you only have time to cook one meal, it should be breakfast.

This is going to get your engine running, providing the energy you need for the day. Plus, if you enjoy a filling meal in the morning, it can help to curb your appetite and reduce cravings throughout the rest of the day. For breakfast, try to enjoy high-protein foods like eggs, oatmeal, or a smoothie with protein powder in it. This is going to get you ready for burning fat all day long.

Mix Up Your Workouts

A common mistake people make when they start exercising more often is doing the same type of workout constantly. If you want to lose weight and burn fat, you need to mix it up. Weight loss plateaus are often the result of eating the same thing, but also doing the same workout. So if you can, try circuit training or at least different types of workouts each week. Add an extra day of weight training or try indoor rock climbing over the weekend instead of going on your normal run. This will work different muscle groups, burning more fat in the long run.

Drink More Cold Water

Not only should you be drinking more water in general, but you should try to drink cold water. The colder the water it is, the higher it raises your metabolism. Keep a pitcher of water in your fridge so you aren't using plastic bottles all day long. This is also a good time for making infused water and keeping the pitcher cold in the refrigerator.

Other Relevant Books by This Author

If you would like to read more relevant books about this topic, here is a list of the Createspace links, titles and descriptions from this author:

https://www.createspace.com/6630449

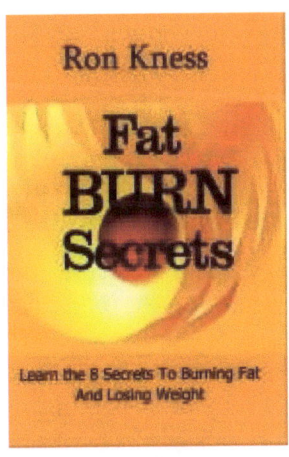

Fat Burn Secrets: Learn the 8 Secrets to Burning Fat and Losing Weight

Now you don't have to blindly spend hours of vigorous training and exercise in the gym anymore.

With this blue print for all exercisers out there, you will discover the importance of this amazing combination: making smart food choices in your daily lifestyle and choosing the right work out for your physical endurance.

Follow the easily learnable techniques in Fat Burn Secrets to obtain optimal results and strip that ugly fat off your body, once and for all.

Topics that Fat Burn Secrets covers include:

- Discover the differences between good fats and bad fats. Learn which unhealthy foods with bad fat that you should avoid and strategize a weight loss diet to lose those extra pounds

- Get fit and healthy with the right mindset. Achieving your ideal body shape takes more than just regular exercise and healthy eating. You need to develop a positive and motivated mind set to keep yourself going

- Find out the ninja secrets behind the slim figure of celebrities and apply the successful methods practiced by them to achieve the body that you've always wanted

- Choose the right cardio workout that suits the physical endurance of your body. Combine low intensity and high intensity cardio workout to strip that fat off your body faster

- Lose weight the right way to avoid the yo-yo effect. Be aware of the causes that can lead to this effect so that you won't regain all the fat that you've previously lost

- Practice yoga as a gentle form of exercise and stress management. If you're a beginner and don't know where to start… Perfect. You can learn all the basics with these easy and relaxing poses

- More fat-inducing foods that you should avoid on a regular basis. Fat Burn Secrets will reveal to you why food flavoring like corn syrup and MSG is hazardous to your health

- Are diet supplements recommended for you? Should you take them? Instead of regularly consuming them, why not try out some alternative ways to eating healthier to ensure your body absorbs all the nutrients that it needs

- Detoxification is now becoming a popular trend among dieters to ultimately burn those excess fats. Learn a variety of detox drinks that will surely give your system a good cleanse like never before

- Getting rid of "Love Handles" has always been a challenging feat. But fret not, because with Fat Burn Secrets' step-by-step exercises, you'll be getting rid of these stubborn fats in no time

- And much more to be uncovered in this fantastic game plan!

To sum it up, you'll learn how to:
- Start feeling energetic and be ready to take on the world!

- Crank your metabolic rate up a few notches

- Burn body fat the right way to reveal toned-looking physique hidden beneath layers of unwanted fat

- Get incredibly shapely hips and thighs and lean, toned abs

Get your copy today; start burning fat tomorrow!

https://www.createspace.com/6880021

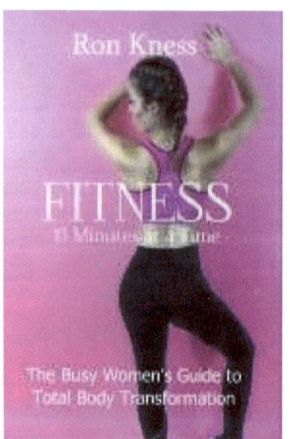

FITNESS - 15 Minutes at a Time: The Busy Women's Guide to Total Body Transformation

We want to be healthier. We also want to be empowered with maintaining our weight and fitness level. And we want to keep the weight off and maintain our healthy lifestyle for the rest of our life!

We can achieve ALL of these goals with the newest release from Ron Kness called *Fitness 15 Minutes at a Time*.

Based on these exciting teachings, you will learn about all the dramatic benefits of getting fit by eating healthy food resulting in weight loss, and doing high intensity exercising.

This book is built around a very clear, concept: improving your appearance and health.

It's not just about getting healthy. Having great fitness level is linked to reducing the risk of many diseases and even reversing the effects of some, such as being overweight and out of shape. These are just two of the many health benefits of being fit and at a normal weight.

In this book, we look at all the ways you can improve your own fitness level, starting with making the decision to get lose weight and healthy. That is the first step - you must want to do it!

This book also looks at the many other steps that can be taken to support this goal, from creating a calorie deficit - burning more calories than you eat - to exercising at a high intensity, to switching to a fitness and weight maintenance mode once at goal . The choices you make about the kind of food you eat and portion sizes has a big impact on your fitness level.

In *Fitness 15 Minutes at a Time*, we'll cover all the bases, giving you everything you need to know to eat healthy, lose weight and get fit.

https://www.createspace.com/6988627

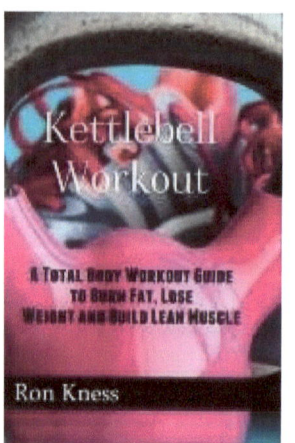

Kettlebell Workout: A Total Body Workout Guide to Burn Fat, Lose Weight and Build Lean Muscle

We want to be functionally stronger - that is building strength that we can use in our everyday lives. We also want to be in charge of our healthy lifestyle. And we want to use kettlebells safely as a workout program!

We can achieve ALL of these goals with the newest release from Ron Kness called *Kettlebell Workout - A Total Body Workout Guide To Burn Fat, Lose Weight And Build Lean Muscle*.

Based on these exciting teachings, you will learn about all the dramatic benefits of using kettlebells as exercise and proper nutrition as a way of getting healthy.

This book is built around a very clear, concept: burn fat, lose weight and build lean muscle.

It's not just about how to use kettlebells to burn fat, lose weight and build lean muscle. Having a great fitness level is linked to making smart exercise and nutrition decisions. This is because people living the healthy lifestyle have learned the value and benefits derived from being healthy.

In this book, we look at all of the ways you can improve your own fitness level, starting with strength training using kettlebells. This book will also look at the many other steps that can be taken to support this goal, from learning how to properly lift and swing kettlebells to torching calories from a kettlebell workout. The choices you make about healthy food and strength training has an impact on your fitness level.

In ***Kettlebell Workout - A Total Body Workout Guide To Burn Fat, Lose Weight And Build Lean Muscle***, we'll cover all the bases, giving you everything you need to know to properly use kettlebells as part of an overall fitness program.

About the Author

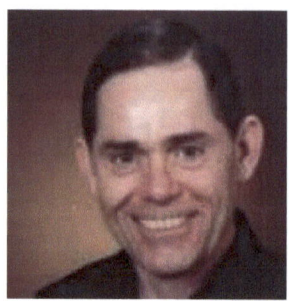

I have published over 125 books on Amazon for Kindle, CreateSpace and other publishing platforms.

While most of my books are on health and fitness in general, as I age (now 65) at the time of this writing) my topics of interest are geared toward aging baby boomers and older.

Besides my own writing, I also ghostwrite ebooks, books, reports, articles, blogs and do Kindle conversions for clients on a variety of topics.

Today my wife and I are retired from our careers and live in Gold Canyon, AZ. I now write as a retirement business where you'll find me happily sitting in my office typing away on my laptop as I work on my next book or ghostwriting project . . . that is if we are not traveling on a cruise ship - our new-found mode of travel.